Nursing & Health Survival Guide

Dental Nursing

Mary Miller

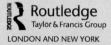

Routledge
Taylor & Francis Group

LONDON AND NEW YORK

First published 2012 by Pearson Education Limited

Published 2014 by Routledge

2 Park Square, Milton Park, Abingdon, Oxon OX14 4RN

711 Third Avenue, New York, NY 10017, USA

Routledge is an imprint of the Taylor & Francis Group, an informa business

Copyright © 2012, Taylor & Francis.

ISBN 13: 978-0-273-75019-2 (hbk)

British Library Cataloguing-in-Publication Data
A catalogue record for this book is available from the British Library

Library of Congress Cataloguing-in-Publication Data
Miller, Mary, 1951-
   Nursing & health survival guide : dental nursing / Mary Miller. -- 1st ed.
       p. ; cm.
   Nursing and health survival guide
   Includes bibliographical references.
   ISBN 978-0-273-75019-2 (pbk.)
   I. Title. II. Title: Nursing and health survival guide.
   [DNLM: 1. Dental Assistants--Great Britain--Handbooks.   2. Dental Care--
methods--Great Britain--Handbooks.   3. Dental Care--nursing--Great Britain--
Handbooks.   4. Dental Instruments--Great Britain--Handbooks.
5. Mouth--Great Britain--Handbooks. WU 49]
   LC Classification not assigned
617.6'0233--dc23

                                                                                    2011047412

Typeset in 8/9.5pt Helvetica by 35

Printed in the UK by Severn, Gloucester on responsibly sourced paper

MIX
Paper from
responsible sources
FSC® C022174

contents

This Survival Guide can be used as a quick reference and also as an aide-memoire. Ideally it can be kept in a pocket for easy use! All members of the dental team will find it useful, so keep a copy in the workplace.

The contents include basic life support, dental charting, definitions and hand washing.

The human skeleton

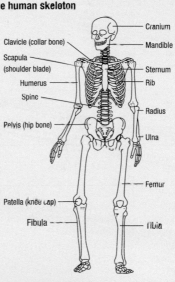

- Cranium
- Clavicle (collar bone)
- Mandible
- Scapula (shoulder blade)
- Sternum
- Humerus
- Rib
- Spine
- Radius
- Pelvis (hip bone)
- Ulna
- Femur
- Patella (knee cap)
- Fibula
- Tibia

Abbreviations

ALARA	As low as reasonably achievable
AOB	Anterior open bite
BPE	Basic periodontal examination
BRA	Bite-raising appliance
CPITN	Community periodontal index of treatment needs
CPD	Continuing professional development
DCP	Dental care professional
EPP	Exposure-prone procedure
GA	General anaesthetic
GDC	General Dental Council
GIC	Glass ionomer cement
HSE	Health and Safety Executive
IRM	Immediate replacement material
LA	Local anaesthetic
NEBDN	National Examining Board for Dental Nurses
NICE	National Institute for Clinical Excellence and Health
PPE	Personal protection equipment
RCT	Root canal treatment
TMJ	Temporomandibular joint
Endo	Prefix meaning within
Intra	Prefix meaning inside, within
Macro	Prefix meaning large
Micro	Prefix meaning small
Dontic	Suffix meaning of the teeth
Ectomony	Complete removal of
Itis	Inflammation of
Otomy	Partial removal of
Peri	Around

Terminology

Anaesthesia	Without feeling
Analgesia	Loss of pain
Abscess	A fluid-filled sac
Abrasion	Wearing away of hard tissue by a physical process, for example toothbrushing
Abutment	Teeth either side of a missing tooth
Anterior	Closer to the front
Apical	Towards the tooth apex
Asepsis	The technique which aims to exclude all microorganisms
Bruxism	Clenching or grinding of teeth
Calculus	Hard deposit of mineralised plaque, also known as tartar
Coronal	Pulp in the crown of a tooth
Decalcification	Loss of calcium which weakens the teeth making them more susceptible to decay
Deep	Further away from the surface
Dentition	Natural teeth in the dental arches
Dentate	Having natural teeth
Edentulous	Having no natural teeth
Erosion	Wearing away of hard tissue by chemical processes, for example by fizzy drinks or acids in fruit
Exfoliate	Natural loss of tooth
Extrinsic	Acting from outside the tooth
Filtrum	Dimple or indentation under the nose directly above the upper lip
Foramen	A natural opening in the bone
Fossa	A depression in the bone

Hyperplasia	Over-development of a tissue
Hypoplasia	Underdevelopment of an organ on tissue
Interproximal	Between teeth
Intrinsic	Acting from inside the tooth
Lateral	To the side
Medial	Closer to the midline of the body
Nausea	Feeling sick
Necrosis	Death of tissue
Osteoblast	Cells which aid the growth and development of teeth and bones
Pathogens	Disease-producing organisms
Periapical	Around the apex of the tooth
Posterior	Closer to the back
Proclined	Sloping in a labial direction
Protrude	Thrust forwards
Retroclined	Leaning backwards
Sinus	An air-filled sac
Radicular	Pulp in the root of the tooth
Superficial	Closer to the surface
Superior	Structures above the surface of other tissues on structures
Supernumerary	An extra tooth in the dentition
Supine	Flat
Xerostomia	Dry mouth

Handwashing technique

Key point

Always wear gloves and remember to wash your hands after removal

Always wear a visor or protective glasses/gloves to prevent aerosol splashback

■ ASEPSIS

In order to aid infection control it is important that aseptic technique is used, and this begins with hand washing.

Hygienic hand washing – five strokes backwards and forwards:

- **Step 1** Palm to palm
- **Step 2** Right palm over back of left hand, left palm over back of right hand
- **Step 3** Palm to palm with fingers interlaced
- **Step 4** Backs of fingers to opposing palm with fingers interlocked
- **Step 5** Rotational rubbing of right thumb clasped over left palm and thumb clasped over right palm
- **Step 6** Rotational rubbing backwards and forwards with clasped fingers of right hand in palm of left hand and clasped fingers of left hand of palm of right hand
- **Step 7** Hands then should be thoroughly rinsed in running water
- **Step 8** Hands then should be thoroughly dried

Hand Hygiene Technique

Decontaminate hands using soap and water using the
following eight steps. Each step consists of five stroke rubbing
backwards and forwards.

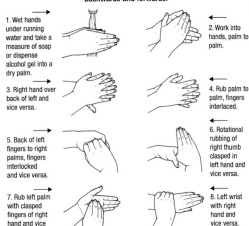

1. Wet hands under running water and take a measure of soap or dispense alcohol gel into a dry palm.

2. Work into hands, palm to palm.

3. Right hand over back of left and vice versa.

4. Rub palm to palm, fingers interlaced.

5. Back of left fingers to right palms, fingers interlocked and vice versa.

6. Rotational rubbing of right thumb clasped in left hand and vice versa.

7. Rub left palm with clasped fingers of right hand and vice versa.

8. Left wrist with right hand and vice versa.

*When using soap and water ensure hands are
thoroughly dry before continuing any task*

Handwashing technique

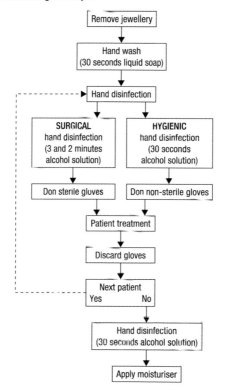

■ HEALTH AND SAFETY AT WORK ACT 1974

The Health and Safety at Work Act 1974 applies to all workplace premises, including dental surgeries. It makes it clear that all employers are responsible not only for the health and safety of their staff but also of anyone who might be on their premises, such as patients or suppliers. All staff and visitors to a workplace should also act in a responsible manner and prevent any hazards occurring that may cause injury to themselves or others.

In addition to the Health and Safety at Work Act 1974, the Dentist's Act 1984 makes the employing dentist accountable for all faults or omissions made by their staff (including dental nurses).

First aid at work

The 1981 Health and Safety (First Aid) Regulations require employers to have suitably trained people to administer first aid to employees who become ill or injured at work.

A first aider is someone who has undergone an approved Health and Safety Executive (HSE) training course in first aid at work.

■ CONTENTS OF THE FIRST AID BOX AS SPECIFIED BY THE HSE

- HSE leaflet on basic advice on first aid at work
- 20 sterile adhesive dressings (assorted sizes)
- 2 sterile eye pads
- 4 triangular bandages
- 6 safety pins

- 6 medium-sized (12 × 12cm) sterile wound dressings
- 2 large (18 × 18cm) sterile unmedicated wound dressings
- 1 pair disposable gloves

The respiratory system

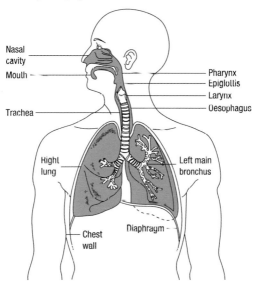

The heart

A diagram of the heart

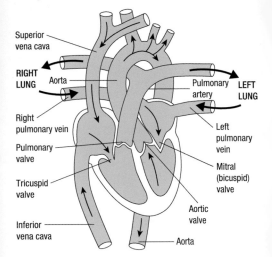

Superior vena cava

RIGHT LUNG

Aorta

Right pulmonary vein

Pulmonary valve

Tricuspid valve

Inferior vena cava

Pulmonary artery

LEFT LUNG

Left pulmonary vein

Mitral (bicuspid) valve

Aortic valve

Aorta

■ CIRCULATION

Left side of the heart Pumps oxygenated blood from the lungs to the rest of the body

Right side of the heart Returns deoxygenated blood from the rest of the body to the lungs

Definitions

RA	Right atrium
RV	Right ventricle
LA	Left atrium
LV	Left ventricle
IVC	Inferior vena cava
SVC	Superior vena cava
TV	Tricuspid valve
MV	Mitral valve

Key point – Circulation

Blood from the head, neck and arms enters the heart via the superior vena cava. Blood from the rest of the body enters the heart from the inferior vena cava travelling from RA – TV – RV – PA to the lungs.

The circulation of deoxygenated blood

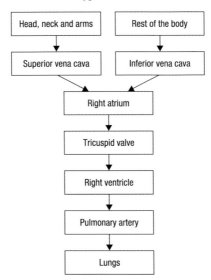

Key point – Circulation

Blood gives up waste carbon dioxide and takes up fresh oxygen – oxygenated blood from the lungs travels through the PV – LA through MV – LV and pumped out by the aorta.

The circulation of oxygenated blood

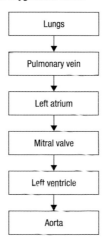

Medical emergencies in the dental surgery

Remember DRABC

Dangers	Assess for electrical, chemical and other dangers
Responsiveness	Shout 'are you alright' and shake patient **CALL FOR HELP**
Airway	Clear and maintain the patient's airway
Breathing	Check breathing (listen and feel) call 999 if necessary
Circulation	Check the carotid pulse, begin cardiac massage if necessary 30 compressions a minute followed by 2 ventilations using an Ambu bag or mask Continue until help arrives **Remember – use up-to-date guidelines**

■ LOCATION OF ESSENTIAL PULSES IN THE HUMAN BODY

The location of pulses in the body

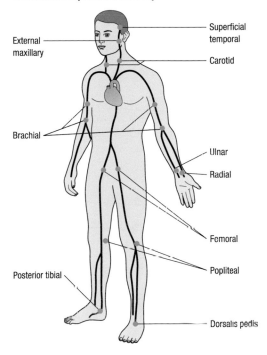

Key point

A pulse is found when an artery crosses a bone.

The periphery pulses are the last to pulsate.

To take a pulse place your first and second fingers over the bone.

Radial pulse   radial bone in the wrist (below thumb)
Carotid pulse   side of the neck level with the Adam's apple
Femoral pulse   top of the leg in the groin

Radial pulse

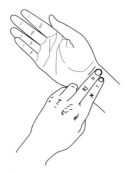

■ FAINTING

The commonest medical emergency in the dental workplace

Signs
- Dizziness
- Weakness
- Light-headedness
- Nausea
- Pallor
- Feels warm but skin cool and clammy
- Slow then rapid pulse
- Loss of consciousness

Treatment
- Call for help
- Lay flat with legs raised to increase the blood flow
- Loosen tight clothing
- Ventilate the area

■ HYPOGLYCAEMIA – COMMON IN DIABETICS

Signs
- Irritable
- Aggressive
- Sweaty skin
- Anxiety
- Tremor
- Confusion
- Disorientation

Treatment
- Call for help
- Give oral glucose or place a sugar lump in the buccal sulcus

■ ANAPHALAXIC SHOCK – AN EXTREME ALLERGIC REACTION, FOR EXAMPLE TO LATEX, NUTS OR ANTIBIOTICS

Signs

- Itchiness
- Weak and rapid pulse
- Low blood pressure
- Wheezing
- Facial swelling
- Cold clammy skin
- Rash
- Collapse

Treatment

- Call for help
- Lay flat with legs raised
- Maintain airway
- Administer 100% oxygen
- Call 999
- Give 1.1000 adrenaline IM (intramuscular)

■ EPILEPTIC FIT

Signs

- Loss of consciousness

Treatment

- Call for help
- Remove any airway obstruction
- Move equipment/objects that may cause harm
- Administer oxygen
- Wait for fit to stop
- If fit continues time the fit
- Call 999
- Continue oxygen

■ MYOCARDIAL INFARCTION

Signs
- Crushing pain in chest and arm
- Paleness
- Sweating
- Nausea
- Rapid weak pulse
- Fast breathing

Treatment
- Call for help
- Clear airway
- Sit the patient upright
- Call 999

■ CARDIAC ARREST

Signs
- Loss of consciousness
- Loss of carotid or femoral pulse
- Fighting for breath
- Dilation of pupils

Treatment
- Call for help
- **SHAKE** patient and **SHOUT** 'Are you alright?'
- Call 999
- Clear and maintain airway
- Commence basic life support (check updated guidelines)

Dental anatomy

The tooth and periodontium

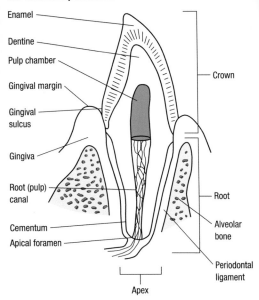

The surfaces of the teeth

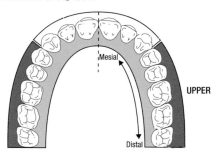

UPPER

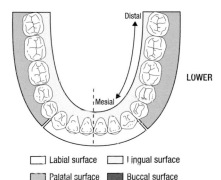

LOWER

☐ Labial surface   ☐ lingual surface

🔲 Palatal surface   ■ Buccal surface

■ SURFACES OF THE TEETH

Mesial	Surface nearest the midline
Distal	Surface furthest away from the midline
Buccal	Surface nearest the cheeks
Labial	Surface nearest the lips
Incisal	Biting edge of the incisors
Occlusal	Biting surface of the premolars and molars
Palatal	Surface nearest the palate
Lingual	Surface nearest the tongue

Deciduous and permanent teeth

Deciduous and permanent teeth

Deciduous teeth

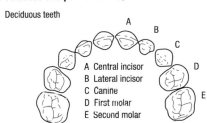

A Central incisor
B Lateral incisor
C Canine
D First molar
E Second molar

Permanent teeth

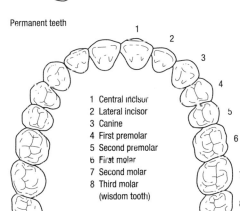

1 Central incisor
2 Lateral incisor
3 Canine
4 First premolar
5 Second premolar
6 First molar
7 Second molar
8 Third molar
(wisdom tooth)

■ DECIDUOUS AND PERMANENT NOTATION

NAMES OF TEETH	DECIDUOUS (28 IF ALL PRESENT)	PERMANENT (32 IF ALL PRESENT)
Central incisor	A	1
Lateral incisor	B	2
Canine	C	3
1st premolar	No premolar	4
2nd premolar	No premolar	5
1st molar	D	6
2nd molar	E	7
3rd molar	No premolar	8

Deciduous and permanent dentition

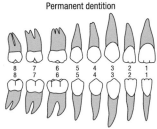

Deciduous dentition   Permanent dentition

■ DIFFERENCES IN DECIDUOUS AND PERMANENT TEETH

DECIDUOUS TEETH
- 20 in the dentition
- White in colour
- Spaces between each tooth
- Bulbous crown
- Larger pulp chamber
- Shorter thin splayed roots
- No premolars
- Smaller overall
- Thinner enamel

PERMANENT TEETH
- 32 in the dentition
- Cream in colour
- Small pulp chamber
- Longer roots

■ DECIDUOUS TEETH ERUPTION DATES

TOOTH	ERUPTION DATES (MAY VARY) MONTHS
A	6
B	8
C	18
D	12
E	24

Deciduous teeth – lower teeth usually erupt before their corresponding upper.

■ PERMANENT TEETH ERUPTION DATES

	ERUPTION DATES (MAY VARY)	
TOOTH	UPPER (YEARS)	LOWER (YEARS)
1	7	7
2	8	8
3	11	9
4	9	10
5	10	11
6	6	6
7	12	12
8	18–24	18–14

■ NUMBER OF ROOTS

Deciduous teeth

TOOTH	NUMBER OF ROOTS (LOWER)	NUMBER OF ROOTS (UPPER)
A	1	1
B	1	1
C	1	1
D	2	3
E	2	3

Permanent teeth

	NUMBER OF ROOTS	
TOOTH	**UPPER**	**LOWER**
1	1	1
2	1	1
3	1	1
4	2 buccal and palatal	1
5	1	1
6	3 mesiobuccal, distobuccal and palatal	2 mesial and distal
7	3 mesiobuccal, distobuccal and palatal	2 mesial and distal
8	3 similar to upper molars	2 mesial and distal

Dental charting

■ REASONS

- Continuity of treatment
- Identification of a body
- In case of legal proceedings

■ ZSIGMONDY–PALMER SYSTEM

The Zsigmondy–Palmer system is frequently used in the United Kingdom.

In the permanent dentition, there are four quadrants which have eight teeth in each (if all present). The permanent teeth are symbolised by the numbers 1 to 8, beginning from the midline. An example of this is the lateral incisors which are referred to as 'upper left 2' (UL2) and 'upper right 2' (UR2). The deciduous teeth are symbolised by the letters A to E, beginning at the midline. An example of this is the lower first molars which are referred to as the 'upper left D' and the 'lower right D'. When recorded, two lines are drawn at right angles to denote the quadrants and the numbers or letters are placed in the quadrant they belong to.

A Zsigmondy–Palmer chart

| 8 | 7 | 6 | 5 | 4 | 3 | 2 | 1 | 1 | 2 | 3 | 4 | 5 | 6 | 7 | 8 |

■ SIGNS AND SYMBOLS

Missing	−
Partially erupted	PE
Unerupted	UE
Recently extracted	X
To be extracted	/
Cavity	o
Temporary dressing	TEMP
Replace restoration	⊙
Restoration present	•
Gold inlay	GI
Porcelain inlay	PI
Preventive resin restoration	PRR
Fissure sealant	FS
Tooth rotated mesially	
Tooth rotated distally	
Tooth drifting	←│→
Tooth missing space closed	→←

Tooth instanding	↓
Tooth outstanding	↓
Retained root	×
Fracture	#
Implant	IMP
Root-filled restoration	RF
	•
Porcelain veneer	PV
Crown	CR
Porcelain bonded crown	PBC
Full gold crown	FGC
Bridge abutment	BA
Bridge pontic	BP
Artificial tooth	A

Roman numerals
I One
II Two
III Three
IV Four
V Five

■ BLACK'S CLASSIFICATION OF CAVITIES AND FILLINGS

Class I   Involving the occlusal surface of the tooth

Class II Involving two or more surfaces of the tooth, for example mesial occlusal, distal occlusal, mesial occlusal distal or extensions, for example mesial occlusal with a palatal extension

Class III Involving the mesial or distal surface of the incisors

Class IV Involving the mesial or distal surface and the biting edge of the incisors

Class V   Involving the gingival third of the tooth, for example palatal, labial, buccal, lingual

■ FDI TWO-DIGIT SYSTEM – THE INTERNATIONAL TOOTH-NUMBERING SYSTEM

Primary teeth

Upper right		Upper left	
55 54 53 52 51		61 62 63 64 65	
85 84 83 82 01		71 72 73 74 75	
Lower right		Lower left	

Permanent teeth

Upper right	Upper left
18 17 16 15 14 13 12 11	21 22 23 24 25 26 27 28
48 47 46 45 44 43 42 41	31 32 33 34 35 36 37 38
Lower right	Lower left

A number replaces the quadrant symbol.

Permanent dentition
Upper right 1
Upper left 2
Lower left 3
Lower right 4

This number identifies the quadrant while the next number identifies the tooth in the quadrant. For example, 11.12.13. is upper right 1, 2 and 3, whereas 31. 32. 33. is lower left 1., 2. and 3.

Deciduous dentition
Upper right 5
Lower left 6
Lower right 7
Upper right 8

For example, 51. 52. 53 is upper right A B C whereas 71. 72. 73. is lower left A, B and C.

Basic periodontal examination (BPE)

CODE	CRITERIA
0	Healthy periodontal tissues – no bleeding after gentle probing
1	Bleeding after gentle probing
	Black band remains completely visible – probing depth up to 3.5mm
	No calculus or defective margins detected
2	Black band remains completely visible – probing depth up to 3.5mm
	Calculus or other plaque-retention factor detected
3	Black band partially visible in deepest pocket – shallow pocket up to 5mm
4	Black band not visible in pocket – deep pocket more than 5.5mm

■ FURCATION INVOLVEMENT

Gingival recession added to probing gives depth of 7mm or more.

The mouth is divided into sextants represented by a single box chart for each sextant. Only the highest score is recorded in each sextant.

Radiographs

A radiograph is a processed film showing an object that has been exposed to X-rays.

Periapical
View   area around the apex of the tooth – root of the tooth
Reason   abscess – root canal treatment – root fracture

Bitewings
View   interproximal (mesial and distal surfaces)
Reason   interproximal caries

Lateral skull
View   side view of the face 1–8 upper and lower
Reason   orthodontic assessment

Orthopantomograph (OPG) and dental panoramic tomograph (DPT)
View   the teeth in all quadrants
Reason   presence, position and pathology of teeth

Pulp testing

The pulp of the teeth either side of the affected tooth is also tested. The patient is asked to raise their hand when they feel a sensation.

■ METHODS

Electric pulp tester (electrical method)
Water or toothpaste is put on the end of the EPT probe to act as a conductor. The probe is placed on the appropriate teeth and a numerical reading will display 0–80 on the pulp tester.

Ethyl chloride (cold method)
Ethyl chloride is sprayed onto a pledget of cotton wool and then placed on the appropriate teeth.

Gutta percha (hot method)
A gutta percha stick is heated and then placed on the appropriate teeth.

Rubber dam

Reasons for using the rubber dam
- Prevent inhalation
- Prevent contamination
- Moisture control
- Enhance visibility
- Patient comfort

Rubber dam equipment

- Rubber dam
- Rubber dam punch to punch a hole through rubber dam sheet
- Rubber dam frame to support the rubber dam
- Rubber dam clamp to keep rubber dam in place
- Rubber dam forcep to hold rubber dam clamp

Orthodontic classification

■ BRITISH STANDARDS INSTITUTE

Incisor relationship

Class I	Lower incisor edge occludes with or below
Class II	Division 1 occlusion upper incisors protrude
Class II	Division 2 occlusion upper central incisors retroclined/tilt backwards
Class III	Occlusion lower incisor edge in front of upper incisors lower jaw forward of upper jaw

Canine relationship

Class I	Tip of upper canine occludes between lower canine and first premolar
Class II	Tip of upper canine occludes between lower lateral incisor and canine
Class III	Tip of upper canine occludes between lower first and second premolar

Molar relationship

Class I	Upper first molar mesial-buccal cusp in buccal groove of lower molar
Class II	Upper first molar mesial cusp is anterior to buccal groove in lower molar
Class III	Upper first molar mesial–buccal cusp is posterior to buccal groove in lower molar

Orthodontic definitions

Overbite	Vertical overlap of the incisor teeth
Overjet	Horizontal distance between labial surface of tips of upper incisors and surface of lower incisors
Anterior open bite	No vertical overlap of lower incisors by upper incisors

Salivary glands

■ PAROTID

One of a pair of glands below and in front of the ear. Stenson's duct runs from it and opens in the mouth opposite the upper second premolar.

■ SUBLINGUAL

The smallest salivary gland in the floor of the mouth which opens on the crest of the sublingual fold under the tongue.

■ SUBMANDIBULAR

One of a pair of glands in the region of the angle which opens on the floor of the mouth beneath the tongue.

Salivary glands

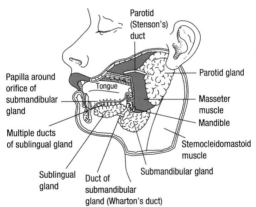

Anatomy of the skull

■ FRONT VIEW OF THE SKULL

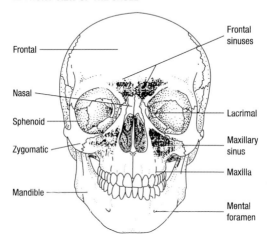

Frontal

Frontal sinuses

Nasal

Lacrimal

Sphenoid

Zygomatic

Maxillary sinus

Maxilla

Mandible

Mental foramen

■ SIDE VIEW OF THE SKULL

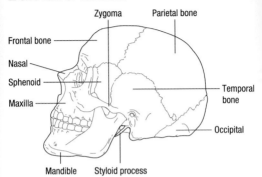

■ BACK VIEW OF THE SKULL

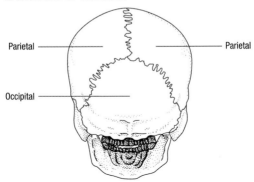

The nerve supply to the teeth and gingivae

■ THE MAXILLA

The maxillary nerve has three branches:
- Anterior superior
- Middle superior
- Posterior superior

NERVE	TEETH ANAESTHETISED	GINGIVAE ANAESTHETISED
Anterior superior	1, 2, 3	Buccal
Middle superior	4, 5, part of 6	Buccal
Posterior superior	part of 6, 7, 8	Buccal
Greater palatine	4, 5, 6, 7, 8	Palate
Long sphenopalatine		Palatal of the incisors canines

Maxillary nerves

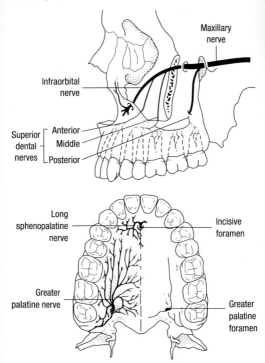

■ THE MANDIBLE

NERVE	SUPPLIES
Inferior dental	All the lower teeth 1–8
Lingual	The lingual gingivae of the lower teeth The anterior two-thirds of the tongue Floor of the mouth
Long buccal	The gingivae of the molars
Mental	The buccal gingivae of the: • Incisors • Canine • Premolars • Lower lip • Chin

Mandibular nerve supply

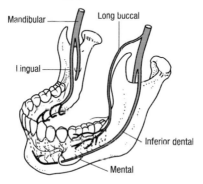

Types of dental injections

- Inferior dental nerve block
- Local infiltration
- Intra-ligamentary

■ INFERIOR DENTAL BLOCK

Site   An inferior dental block is given in the mandibular foramen. As this is close to the lingual nerve, the lingual gingivae and half the tongue are anaesthetised as well. The only part unaffected is the buccal gingivae.

Supplies Anaesthetises the nerve trunk

■ LOCAL INFILTRATION

Site   Above the apex of the tooth to be anaesthetised

Supplies Anaesthetises the nerve endings

■ INTRA-LIGAMENTARY

Site   Directly into the gingival crevice to the periodontal ligament on the mesial and distal sides

Supplies The tooth and the buccal and lingual gingivae

Muscles of mastication

- The fifth cranial nerve or trigeminal nerve
- Optic nerve
- Maxillary nerve
- Mandibular nerve

	ORIGIN	INSERTION	ACTION
Lateral pterygoid	Behind the maxilla	Condyle	Pulls the mandible forward and swings it to the opposite side
Medial pterygoid	Behind the maxilla	Inside the ramus of the mandible	Closes the mandible
Masseter	Zygomatic arch	Outside the ramus	Closes the mandible
Temporalis	Temporal fossa (side of the head)	Coronoid process	Closes and pulls the mandible backwards

The temporal muscle

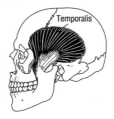

The masseter muscle

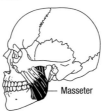

Lateral and medial pterygoid muscle

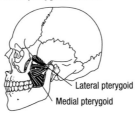

Muscles of facial expression

Key point

Bell's Palsy affects the seventh cranial nerve (facial nerve).
A stroke can affect the buccinator muscle.

	SITE	ACTION
Buccinator	Cheek	Used when chewing food
Orbicularis oculi	Around the eye	
Orbicularis oris	Around the lips and mouth	Used when playing a brass instrument

The muscles of facial expression

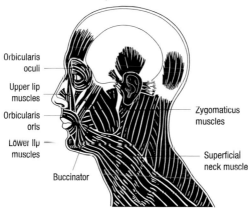

Orbicularis oculi

Upper lip muscles

Orbicularis oris

Lower lip muscles

Buccinator

Zygomaticus muscles

Superficial neck muscle

Handpieces

■ AIROTA
- Standard or miniature head
- Friction grip burs

■ CONTRA-ANGLED
- Latch grip burs
- Mandrels
- Polishing brushes/cups

■ STRAIGHT
- Straight burs
- Surgical burs
- Acrylic trimmers

Burs

■ STANDARD
- Adults and children

Ends
- Friction grip
- Latch grip
- Straight

■ MINIATURE
- To treat adults who are unable to open their mouth wide
- To gain access to the third molars (wisdom teeth) at the back of the mouth
- To treat children

Shank
- Stainless steel

■ HEAD

Diamond (cutting)
- Uncut, rough to touch (coarse–medium)
- Used to remove enamel, amalgam and composite

Diamond (finishing)
- Smooth finish (fine–superfine)
- Used to remove excess material, smooth and shape composite restoration

Tungsten carbide (cutting)
- Smooth to touch and shines in the light
- Used to remove enamel, amalgam and composite

Tungsten carbide (finishing)
- Smooth finish
- Used to remove excess composite material, smooth, shape composite restoration

Carbon steel
- Dull-coloured
- Used to remove dentine, caries

Finishing burs – tungsten carbide

Round

Flame

Bullet

Needle

Tapered
fissure

Diamond-cutting burs

Round

Pear

Inverted cone

Diablo

Carbon steel burs

Round

Inverted cone

Flat fissure

Shape
- Flat fissure
- Tapered fissure
- Round
- Pear
- Inverted cone
- Diablo

Hand pieces
- Airota
- Contra-angled
- Straight

Mandrels

Mandrels

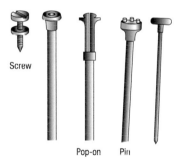

Screw

Pop-on   Pin

Latch grip and straight
- Inserted into a contra-angled or straight hand piece
- Used in conjunction with paper, sandpaper and other discs to smooth and shape

Moore's mandrel
- The disc is placed on the diamond-shaped middle

Pop-on mandrel
- The disc is popped on to the circular-shaped middle

Screw-on mandrel
- The disc goes between the screw and the mandrel is then screwed into the shank

Pin mandrel
- The pin goes through the middle of the disc and then slides back into the shank

Extraction forceps

■ DECIDUOUS FORCEPS

Lower molars

Lower roots and centrals

Upper centrals

Upper roots and centrals

Upper bicuspids

■ UPPER PERMANENT FORCEPS

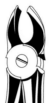

Right side
Upper right molar

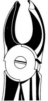

Left side
Upper left molar

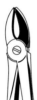

Upper roots

Upper straight

■ LOWER PERMANENT FORCEPS

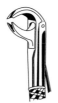

Lower molar
split-beak

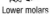

Lower molars

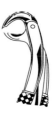

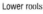

Lower roots

Elevators

- Warwick James
- Cryers

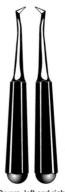

Cryers, left and right

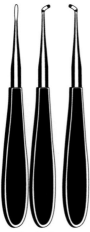

Warwick James
straight, left and right

Chisels

Couplands chisels

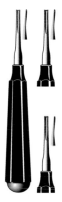

Post-operative instructions

INSTRUCTIONS	REASONS
Do not rinse your mouth for 12 hours	This will wash away the blood clot and cause a reactionary haemorrhage
Do not drink hot liquids or alcohol for the rest of the day	Hot liquids can burn the soft tissue and may dislodge the blood clot. Alcohol will raise the blood pressure, which will disturb the clot and cause bleeding
Do not do any physical work or exercise for the rest of the day	Exercise will raise the blood pressure and cause bleeding
Eat or drink on the other side of your mouth	As your lip or cheek or both are numb
Take normal painkillers if necessary	
The following day rinse your mouth with a warm salty mouthwash using one teaspoon of salt in a tumbler of warm water. Do this three to four times a day for at least two days	This will encourage healing
Brush your teeth as normal, being careful to avoid the treated area	
If bleeding occurs sit down and bite on a folded tissue for 20 minutes	This should stop the bleeding

If bleeding still persists or you are worried following your treatment, contact the surgery. If the surgery is closed contact the emergency number on the appointment card or go to your doctor or accident and emergency department.

Other reading

Dental Nursing Monthly	www.dental-nursing.co.uk
Mosby's Textbook of Dental Nursing	Miller and Scully, Elsevier
Advanced Dental Nursing	Robert Ireland, Blackwell/Munksgaard
Harty's Dental Dictionary	Heasman and McCracken, Elsevier

Useful contacts

National Examining Board for Dental Nurses
110 London Street
Fleetwood
Lancashire FY7 6EU
Tel: 01253 778417
Website: www.nebdn.org

British Association of Dental Nurses
PO Box 4, Room 200
Hillhouse International Business Centre
Thornton Cleveleys   F75 4QD
Tel: 0870 2110113
Website: www.badn.org.uk

BADN National Education Group (BADN NEG)
PO Box 4, Room 200
Hillhouse International Business Centre
Thornton Cleveleys
F75 4QD

General Dental Council
37 Wimpole Street
London W1G 8DO
Tel: 0845 2224141
Email: dcp@gdc-uk.org
Website: www.gdc-uk.org

Society for the Advancement of Anaesthesia in Dentistry (SAAD)
www.saaduk.org

National Oral Health Promotion Group (NOHPG)
Website: www.nohpg.org

British Society of Dental and Maxillofacial Radiology
Website: www.bsdmfr.org.uk

Society and College of Radiographers
207 Providence Square
Mill Street
London SE1 2EW
Tel: 020 7740 7200
Website: www.sor.org

British Orthodontic Society
291 Gray's Inn Road
London WC1X 8QF
Tel: 020 7837 2193
Website: www.bos.org.uk

British Society for Disability and Oral Health (BSDH)
Website: www.bsdh.org.uk